Stretchin

The Top 100 Best Stretches of All Time

Increase Flexibility, Gain Strength, Relieve Pain & Prevent Injury!

By Ace McCloud
Copyright © 2016

Disclaimer

The information provided in this book is designed to provide helpful information on the subjects discussed. This book is not meant to be used, nor should it be used, to diagnose or treat any medical condition. For diagnosis or treatment of any medical problem, consult your own physician. The publisher and author are not responsible for any specific health or allergy needs that may require medical supervision and are not liable for any damages or negative consequences from any treatment, action, application or preparation, to any person reading or following the information in this book. Any references included are provided for informational purposes only. Readers should be aware that any websites or links listed in this book may change.

Table of Contents

Introduction 6

Chapter 1: The Many Benefits of Stretching 8

Chapter 2: How to Stretch Properly 10

Chapter 3: Warming Up 15

Chapter 4: Leg Stretches 18

Chapter 5: Arm and Shoulder Stretches 23

Chapter 6: Back Stretches 28

Chapter 7: Hip Stretches 32

Chapter 8: Neck 37

Chapter 9: Chest 40

Chapter 10: Hands 42

Chapter 11: Full Body Stretches 45

Chapter 12: Sample Stretching Routines 47

Chapter 13: Creating Your Own Stretching Routine 58

Conclusion 61

My Other Books and Audio Books 62

DEDICATED TO THOSE WHO ARE PLAYING THE GAME OF LIFE TO

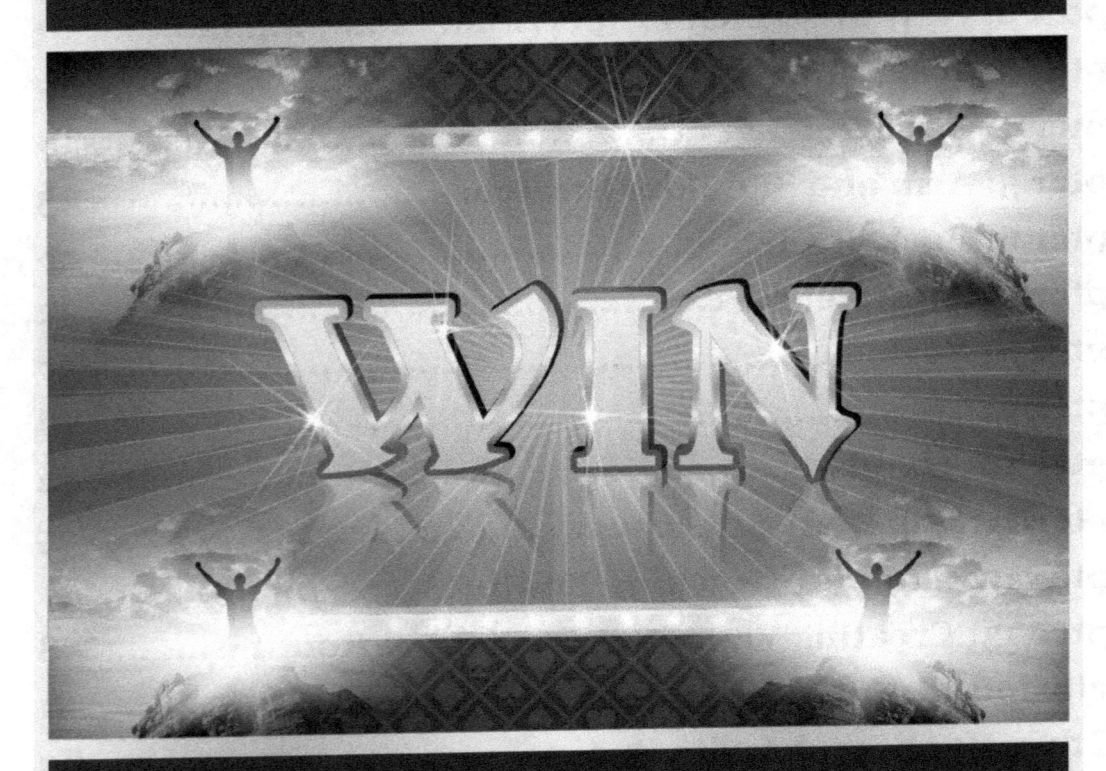

WIN

KEEP ON PUSHING AND NEVER GIVE UP!

Ace McCloud

Be sure to check out my website for all my Books and Audio books.

www.AcesEbooks.com

Introduction

I want to thank you and congratulate you for buying the book, "Stretching: The Top 100 Best Stretches Of All Time: Increase Flexibility, Gain Strength, Relieve Pain & Prevent Injury."

Stretching – everyone has heard of it, but is it possible that we don't understand just how truly important it is? To stretch is to literally to lengthen your muscles. Stretching is often performed before exercising or when preparing to play a sport or perform in a competition. However, stretching is much more important than many people think; it can proactively prevent injuries, heal past injuries, and help to maintain a healthy and balanced body.

You probably had your first introduction to stretching the same way I did, during gym class at school. However, now that I have written this book, I've come to conclude that the basics of stretching we received in gym class is just a touch of its actual greatness. If today's teachers and coaches are still starting class cold with stretching and ending it without, they are shortchanging their students.

I am so glad you've chosen to read this book, because you will now discover what stretching is all about. The truth is, the human body is very complex; each part of our bodies has unique muscles designed for specific purposes. Each of our muscle groups can benefit from stretching and over time a regular stretching routine gives tremendous overall life benefits.

There is no way you can stretch every muscle group optimally in a single 40-minute class period; if you intend to gain the true benefits of stretching, you will need to pursue it on your own time, for yourself. This book contains proven steps and strategies that will help you design a stretching routine that works best for you.

In the pages that follow, you will discover the amazing benefits of stretching and learn what happens when you neglect it! This book contains stretches that cover each major part of your body. You will learn the four basic types of stretches and receive full instructions in stretching out your entire body. You'll also discover how to stretch properly and how to keep committed to your routine. You'll discover the importance of warming up and will learn how to design a basic warm-up routine to get your body ready for stretching. Finally, you'll be provided with some sample stretching routines, ranging from beginning to advanced levels and by the end of this book you'll know how to create your own stretching routine – one that fits your schedule and your specific needs!

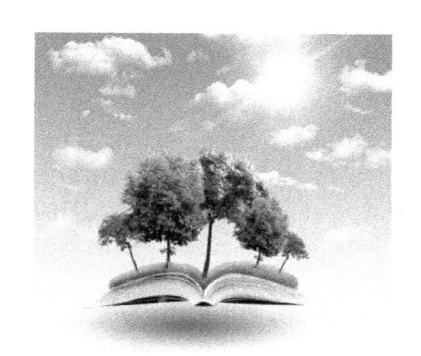

Chapter 1: The Many Benefits of Stretching

Stretching is a basic and instinctive action that people often engage in automatically. How many times have you stretched after waking up or after sitting in the same position for a long time? Although basic stretching comes naturally, its health benefits when practiced deliberately are not very well-known.

Incorporating a full stretching routine into your day is just as important for maintaining a strong, healthy body as is a workout routine. Stretching comes with many benefits, including:

- Maximized flexibility and range of motion throughout your body
- The prevention of muscle strains
- The ability to use everyday motions with minimal discomfort
- The ability to lead an active lifestyle
- Improved balance and coordination
- Improved posture
- Improved skeletal alignment
- The prevention of injuries
- The reduction of muscle soreness
- Faster healing of injuries
- Improved ability to handle stress, minimizing effects of stress on your body
- Improved circulation
- Improved coordination

What Happens When You Don't Stretch?

If you do not stretch your muscles adequately, the most obvious result is increased stiffness and soreness in your muscles. When your muscles are stretched and relaxed regularly, they are able to smoothly slide over other body parts, giving your body a full range of motion. However, when your muscles have not been made flexible through stretching, they begin to form fibers that gradually grow denser and denser. When the fibers grow too thick, due to a lack of movement, your range of motion becomes impaired.

It is important to remember that while stretching is important, over-stretching can cause permanent damage to your tendons. While a muscle can stretch to nearly one and a half times its length, a tendon cannot be stretched beyond 4% of its length. To prevent possible damage to your tendons, most experts recommend that you hold a stretch no longer than 60 seconds.

Stretching is recommended for people of every age. It is especially important for children to stretch so that their muscles and joints will remain flexible as they develop into adulthood. Adults also need to stretch to retain full range of motion and to minimize bone loss as they age; for them, stretching is preventative medicine.

There is a myth that you eventually grow too old to stretch, but that's far from the truth. Not only can stretching improve your ability to safely and efficiently use different parts of your body as you age, but it's a perfect way to relax and clear your mind, especially for busy people.

My life is so hectic and full of responsibility that I never thought I'd have time to incorporate a relaxing, therapeutic activity into my life. Yet, when I discovered stretching my whole life changed. I either prepare myself for the day ahead of me by stretching, right after I drink my morning cup of coffee (that *really* puts me in a positive mood!), or I use it to unwind after a long, stressful day. When I stretch, I usually start by starting up some favorite music, grabbing a couple small pieces of equipment, and then warming up into my personal stretching routine.

To learn more about the benefits and practicality of stretching, check out the YouTube testimonial by a doctor who discovered the benefits of stretching as he aged: Being Flexible: Benefits of Stretching | Dr. Weston by Sunwarrior.

Stretching comes naturally for humans. As I mentioned in the introduction, you may have caught yourself stretching instinctively after sitting in the same position for a long time. Stretching does not require any special training beyond what you may learn in this book. It's incredibly easy and can be done almost anywhere, if you have a little imagination! It's so easy to do that I have to ask, "How could anyone NOT learn to stretch?"

Chapter 2: How to Stretch Properly

Like any kind of exercise, stretching comes with a basic set of rules that you should follow to ensure that you're doing it properly and safely. Overstretching – or overworking – your muscles can lead to damage that can hinder your everyday performance and may cause permanent damage that costs you in opportunities, medical bills, and in your range of motion. In this chapter, you will discover the do's and don'ts of stretching so that you can easily stretch your muscles without worrying about hurting yourself and having to take time off to recover.

There are four categories of stretching: **dynamic, ballistic, static,** and **isometric.**

Dynamic stretching occurs when you move throughout the stretch. You use the momentum of your body to stretch your muscles. This is most common with sport-specific movements. One example of a dynamic stretch is arm circles. Research shows that dynamic stretching is best for preventing muscle tightness, which is often correlated with muscle tear injuries.

If you're an athlete, this is the best type of stretching to use to warm up before competition because it helps utilize the momentum of athletic forms and decreases your risk of injury while you are playing. Dynamic stretching should be done slowly and with care, as sudden movements can push you beyond your range of motion and increase your chances of injury.

Ballistic stretching is a form of dynamic stretching that incorporates a bouncing motion as part of the stretch. The purpose is to stress your muscles farther, before they have a chance to relax. Recent research has shown that ballistic stretching can cause muscle tightness, making a person increasingly susceptible to injuries. As a result, stretching experts often shy away from this stretching category. We will not include ballistic stretching in this book.

Static stretching involves holding a single position to promote maximum flexibility. An example is when you stretch out one of your legs on the floor and stretch your arms toward your toes for a set number of seconds. Static stretching can help gradually increase your range of motion. Static stretching can also increase protection against movement-related injuries. For athletes, static stretching promotes an increased production of force, improved jumping height, and greater speed.

There are two sub-types of static stretching: **static passive** and **static active** stretching. In static passive stretching you use an external resource to hold your stretch, such as your hand or a towel. This type of stretching is helpful for soothing muscle spasms, cooling down after a workout or healing injuries.

Static active stretching occurs when you use the strength of your opposing muscles to hold a stretch. For example, standing on one leg and extending the other to stretch it is a static active stretch. This type of stretching promotes active flexibility. Static active stretches should be held for a minimum of 10 seconds and no longer than 30 seconds. Athletes should avoid static active stretches before a competition, as they can result in balance impairment and a reduction in force.

Isometric stretching promotes static passive flexibility. Many people who practice karate and martial arts are familiar with isometric stretching. Because this type of stretching is so extreme, it is very important that those who engage in it approach it with caution. Many static passive stretches can easily turn into an isometric stretch. For example, if you stretch out your leg on a bench using your own weight to hold the stretch and then you contract your leg muscles by trying to bend your knee, you are performing an isometric stretch. When you increase tension in a muscle without changing its length, you are creating an isometric contraction.

Since isometric stretching is very complex and must be approached with caution, there are a few important guidelines you must follow to ensure that these stretches benefit your body. First, you should always leave at least two days in between an isometric stretching routine. As with weightlifting, your muscles need time to recover from this type of exercise.

When stretching, perform a single stretch per muscle group in each session and limit each stretch to a maximum of 5 sets with a minimum of 2 per set. You should only hold each stretch for a maximum of 15 seconds.

Spend about 10 minutes doing light warm-up exercises before you begin these stretches. Aerobic exercises and dynamic stretching will suffice as a warm-up. Finally, experts recommend that anybody under the age of 18 should not engage in isometric stretching.

Stretching Basics

Every stretching routine differs, but there are some universal basics you should follow to ensure you're off to a good start and are stretching properly. By following these basics, you will increase your chances of successfully becoming flexible:

1. **Always Warm Up First** – Warming up before you start stretching your muscles is very important. If you try to stretch cold muscles, you increase your chances of injury. Warming up gets your blood flowing to your tissues so that your muscles are more protected when you do stretch. Your warm up does not need to be elaborate; you only need to engage in a light aerobic activity, such as jogging or walking, and then only for 5 to 10 minutes.

2. **Start With Dynamic Stretches** – After you warm up, it is best to start your routine with dynamic stretches. Since dynamic stretches consist of slow, controlled movements, they can also help you continue to warm up while stretching at the same time. If you're preparing to stretch before a workout or competition, starting with dynamic stretches is also very beneficial.
3. **Move on to Static Stretches** – After you perform some dynamic stretches, you can move on to your workout or competition or just go directly to static stretches to improve your muscle length and flexibility.
4. **Focus on Your Sport** – If you are an athlete looking to develop a stretching routine, it is important to include the types of stretches that are specifically beneficial to the sport you play. Incorporating sport-specific stretches into your routine can help prevent sports related injuries.
5. **Do Not Overstretch** – Never stretch your muscles to the point that they become painful. Dynamic stretching should never induce pain. Static stretching should bring on some discomfort but it should never be enough to make you wince.

How Long Should You Hold a Stretch?

Different types of static stretches require different holding times, and dynamic stretches aren't held at all. Knowing the proper holding time for a stretch is very important to avoid overstretching injuries. Stretch times differ, based on your experience level.

Experts recommend that an effective static stretch be held for no longer than 30 seconds. Beginners may find it difficult to hold a stretch for 30 seconds because their bodies are not accustomed to this level of stretching. Most beginners should start out by holding a stretch for 10 seconds, then increasing the time as the stretch becomes easier. It is important to remember that complex stretches, such as isometric stretches, should also only be held for 10 to 15 seconds despite your experience level. Even when you've achieved an advanced stretching level, you should never push yourself beyond 30 seconds. Doing so could result in an injury.

The YouTube video, <u>How Long to Hold a Stretch</u> by Mark Rosenberg, D.C. provides some great insight on stretch times.

More Tips on Stretching:

- It is a common misconception that people should engage in static stretching before a workout. While static stretching can help you maintain flexibility, *and should* be included in a separate stretching routine, it is *actually* best to engage in this type of stretching *after* a workout.

Cooling down your muscles with a few post-workout static stretches can help reduce the chances that your muscles will be sore the next day. As long as you stick to a consistent stretching routine, you should not need to stretch before a workout because your routine will already have promoted flexibility.

- Use a tool such as a resistance band or a pull-up bar to provide traction when you're stretching. This can help increase your range of motion while preventing joint impingement.

- Start out by stretching slowly. If you're a beginner, you're not going to have full range of motion right away. For example, if you're a beginner doing toe touches, your fingers will probably not reach your feet right away. Begin by performing a comfortable stretch until you can push yourself to the next level. Pushing yourself too far too soon can lead to an injury.

- Don't allow poor posture to prevent you from engaging in a stretching routine. In fact, it is especially important to stretch if your posture isn't up to par. Poor posture often occurs because your muscles have contracted, growing shorter over time. Increasing your range of motion can lead to improved posture and an overall feeling of well-being.

- Before you start stretching, analyze your body for any tight muscles and work on stretching those first. The tight muscles can limit your ability to perform full range-of-motion exercises in other parts of your body.

- <u>Don't</u> stretch the minute you jump out of bed. Your spine fills up with fluid while you sleep so stretching immediately after waking up dramatically increases your chances of injuring yourself. Wait at least one hour before you start stretching.

- Avoid contracting a muscle immediately after you have worked on stretching it.

- Continue to breathe normally. Never hold your breath while stretching; doing so will cause your muscles to tense up. Focus on taking more time to exhale than on your inhale. This will help your muscles remain relaxed as you stretch, minimizing your chances of injury.

- Focus on building balance in flexibility between front and back as well as left and right. For example, if you have one tight hamstring, focus on stretching it until both of your hamstrings feel evenly stretched.

Finding the Motivation to Stretch

Stretching is an important activity that you should incorporate into your daily life, but like any other repeated activity it can become boring or feel tedious at times. Some days you may feel tempted to shorten your routine or skip stretching altogether. Finding the motivation to stretch consistently can prevent you from losing any physical gains made so far and from losing a hard-won good habit.

Unlike most traditional exercise, stretching does not require a special environment or equipment. If you consistently engage in another static activity, such as watching TV at a certain time each night, you can always stretch while you watch, thus getting two tasks done at once. It also helps to find a stretching buddy, someone to stretch with. Stretching with a friend or family member can help you keep accountable to stretch regularly. A stretching buddy also gives you someone to talk with as you stretch, helping your muscles stay relaxed, distracting you from discomfort, and making the time pass more quickly.

Another effective motivator is knowing your "why." Why is stretching important to you? A common answer is to because you want to feel good about yourself. A close second is the desire to avoid injury, whether you're an athlete or a "regular Joe."

As an athlete, a powerful motivator is to visualize your life as if you were injured and no longer able to play the sport you love. In contrast, whether you're an athlete or a "normal" person, just imagining how good it will feel to be flexible and less-prone to injury may be motivation enough.

Make stretching something you look forward to. Whether or not you're an athlete, we are all human. Sometimes it's a relief to spend a half hour or so of quiet in the midst of your day, stepping away for a moment from all the stresses and sheer busyness of life. Turn your stretching routine into a relaxing activity that can help you re-balance and refresh your mind. I look forward to my stretching time every day because I know it will clear my mind and nurture my spirit while strengthening my body.

Chapter 3: Warming Up

Prior to this chapter, I discussed how important it is to warm up before you begin your stretching routine. Though experts in the past have recommended stretching before a workout, they are beginning to lean more towards recommending stretches following a workout. Why? The answer is simply because cold muscles should never be stretched. Cold muscles aren't as loose as warm muscles and by stretching before a warm up, your chances of pulling a muscle are dramatically increased. Your warm-up routine does not have to be elaborate and only needs to last up to 10 minutes.

Warming up brings several benefits to your body. First, it increases the amount of blood flow to your heart and other muscles, which helps prepare them for an extra work load. It also increases the amount of oxygen and nutrients that are sent to your muscles. The increased aerobic activity prevents you from easily becoming out of breath. In addition, it lubricates your joints. Finally, warming up can also help you mentally prepare for your stretching routine; it boosts your energy levels and helps pump up your enthusiasm.

To start your warm up you want to engage in **light aerobics**. This could include taking a brisk walk, a slow jog, or a quick spin on a stationary bike. You could also march in place, walk up and down a flight of stairs, bounce on a mini trampoline, take a swim or engage in any activity that gets your heart pumping.

Dynamic Stretches

Roller Recovery: If you discover that any particular muscles are tight after your warm-up, you can run a foam roller over those spots for 10 to 30 seconds and then hold the muscles in a static stretch for 30 seconds. This should help loosen them up and return them to their normal length before you proceed with dynamic stretching.

A light dynamic stretching routine will continue to warm up your muscles even as you stretch them. Here is a good dynamic warm up routine:

Note: when a description below mentions only one side of your body, perform it on the other side as well. Your objective is to reach balanced flexibility

Prisoner Squats: Stand with your feet slightly farther apart than your shoulders. Place your hands behind your head. Lower your body into a squat and look upward. Squat down as far as possible without bending your knees any further. Hold that position for a moment and then push yourself back up. For additional force building, you can propel yourself up off the ground when you push back up if you choose.

Jump Rope: Rapidly jump up and down while quickly twirling a jump rope underneath your feet. Spring up from the ground using primarily your feet and ankles.

Jumping Jacks: Stand with your feet together and your arms at rest by your sides. Keeping both arms and legs relatively straight, jump up while widening your stance and raising your arms away from your sides to clap your hands over your head. Jump up a second time, returning both feet and hands to their original position Repeat this motion without pause until you feel your heart pumping.

Ankle Bounces: Rapidly jump and up and down, springing off the floor with your feet and ankles.

Walking Lunges: Stand tall with your feet shoulder width apart. Step forward into a lunge and bend both knees to lower your hips to the ground. Avoid touching your back knee to the ground. Shift your weight onto your forward foot and use your back foot to push off the ground; bring your back leg forward and step into another lunge.

Side Step Lunge: Stand upright with your feet slightly apart and your knees slightly bent. Keeping your left knee and toes aligned above each other, step directly to your left. With your weight shifted onto the left leg, bring your right foot toward the left until you have returned to the starting posture. This may be repeated to the left, then performed to the right the same number of times.

Toe Touches: Stand upright with your feet shoulder distance apart. Bend at the waist, allowing your arms to hang downwards as you lower your upper body headfirst. Relax and allow your arms and torso to naturally hang in front of your legs. Allow your body to hang and relax for 20 seconds.

Power Skips: Skip rapidly as high and as far forward as you can.

Arm Circles: Stand upright with your legs shoulder distance apart, holding your arms out to each side, palms facing forward. Slowly begin swinging your arms in small circles as you breathe normally. Move your arms in a circular motion for at least ten seconds; then, rest them a few minutes and repeat the exercise, making circles in the opposite direction.

Crunches: lie on your back on the floor. Place your hands together behind your head. Without bending your neck, raise your torso until your shoulder blades come up off the floor. Lower yourself to the starting position and repeat multiple times.

Lateral Leg Swings: Stand and face a wall, touching it with your hands as needed for balance. Lift your left foot about an inch off the ground. Swing the left leg out (to the left) and back about 10 times. Put your left foot down and repeat the process with your right leg.

Pendulum Swings: Stand a couple feet behind a chair back with your legs shoulder width apart. Keeping a straight back and bending your knees slightly, lean forward at the waist and grasp the top of the chair with your right hand. Let your left arm hang loose from the shoulder socket. Using your upper body to start the motion, swing the left arm back and forth, both from side to side, front to back, and in a circular motion, about 10 times each. Then, repeat this exercise with your right arm.

Shoulder Rolls: While seated on a chair, rest your hands on your legs. Breathe in and roll your shoulders backward, up, forward and down as you breathe out. Let your shoulders rest, then take another deep breath in and roll your shoulders the opposite direction as you breathe out.

Run in Place: Run in place, lifting your knees high. Perform this warm-up for one minute.

Single Leg Hops: Stand on your left leg, behind a marker of some sort. Flex your knee, then jump forward over the marker, landing on your left leg. You can set up multiple markers for a multiple-hop exercise if you want. Remember to repeat on the right leg.

Standing Hip Circles: Balance on your left leg, with your right hand holding onto something for support. Raise your right knee up to a 90 degree angle and draw a circle in the air with it. This allows you to open up your hips. Draw a circle in the opposite direction, then repeat with the right leg.

Paulwebb.tv has put together a video containing a really good stretching warm up routine, called [Full Body Dynamic Warm Up](); it will demonstrate most of these exercises,

Chapter 4: Leg Stretches

Your legs, which contain your quadriceps, hamstring and gluteal muscles are an important part of your body. Without your legs, you wouldn't be able to walk, climb, jump or otherwise easily transport yourself. Tight leg muscles are a common problem among humans, largely because the majority of us sit for most of the day. When your knees are bent, the muscles that flex the joint in your knee shorten, creating tightness. Not only can tight leg muscles increase your chances of an injury but they are often a cause of back pain. Since you will need top-of-the-line legs for the duration of your life, performing leg stretches on a daily basis can loosen tight muscles and prevent both pain and injuries.

Note: when a description below mentions only one side of your body, perform it on the other side as well. Your objective is to reach balanced flexibility

Standing Quadriceps Stretch
Level: Beginner
Stretch Time: 10-30 seconds

Stand straight with your right hand against a wall for support; then, bend your left foot behind you. Take your left hand and pull your heel to your buttocks. Stand straight and continue to pull your foot up until you feel the stretch in your thigh.

Side Quadriceps Stretch
Level: Beginner
Stretch Time: 10-30 seconds

Lie down on your left side. Bring the calf of your right leg back until your knee sticks out and you feel the stretch in your thigh.

Prone Quadriceps Stretch
Level: Beginner
Stretch Time: 10-30 seconds

Lie on your stomach and stretch out your legs straight behind you. Lift your left leg off the floor until only your knee makes contact it and you can feel the stretch in your quads. Repeat this with the right leg.

Hamstring Stretch
Level: Beginner
Stretch Time: 10-30 seconds

Lie on your back and bend your knees. Lift one leg and slightly bend your knee while pulling on the back of your upper leg until it is at 90-degrees. Once your knee is in this angle, straighten your knee out until the back of your leg stretches fully.

Hamstring Variation #1
Level: Beginner
Stretch Time: 10-30 seconds

Sit on the floor and stretch your legs out in front of you. Keeping your knees straight, reach your arms forward as you bend at your waist.

Hamstring Variation #2
Level: Beginner
Stretch Time: 10-30 seconds

Sit on the floor with your legs before you in a V position. Bend your left leg until you can place the sole of your foot against your right leg. Reach your arms forward over your right leg by bending forward at your waist.

Hamstring Variation #3
Level: Beginner
Stretch Time: 10-30 seconds

Stand straight with your feet shoulder width apart. Cross your left foot over the right. Bend at your waist and slowly lower your head to your front knee while keeping both knees straight. Straighten up and repeat the stretch with your right foot crossed over the left.

Hamstring Variation #4
Level: Beginner
Stretch Time: 10-30 seconds

Stand facing a wall, about one foot away from it. Push your hands into the wall and take one step back with your left foot. With a straight back, press your left heel into the ground and allow your left hamstring to stretch.

Calf Stretch
Level: Beginner
Stretch Time: 10-30 seconds

Stand facing a wall. Lean in toward the wall, placing your hands on it for support, without moving your legs or feet and keeping your knees and waist straight. Make sure your heels stay in contact with the ground as you lean into the wall until a stretch occurs in your calves.

Calf Stretch Variation #1
Level: Beginner
Stretch Time: 10-30 seconds

Sit down and stretch out your legs in front of you. Hold a towel with one end in each hand. Pull your toes inward by placing the towel around the ball of your feet.

Calf Stretch Variation #2
Level: Beginner
Stretch Time: 10-30 seconds

Stand facing a wall, one step behind it. Step forward with your left leg. Pressing your right heel into the ground, lower your body and keep your back leg straight as you lean against the wall. Lower yourself until you can feel a stretch.

Calf Stretch Variation #3
Level: Beginner
Stretch Time: 10-30 seconds

Stand facing a wall. Bend the toes of your left foot up the base of the wall while your heel touches the ground. Point your toes up until the stretch occurs. Return to your starting position and repeat for your right leg.

Butterfly Stretch
Level: Beginner
Stretch Time: 10-30 seconds

This stretch will work your inner thighs, your hip flexors and your groin. Sit down and cross your legs Indian style. Bring the soles of your feet together. Slowly push your thighs open by pressing down on them with your arms. You can lean forward for a more advanced stretch if you wish.

Glute Stretch
Level: Beginner
Stretch Time: 10-30 seconds

This stretch targets your gluteal muscles, which helps your body with leg extension and rotation. Lie on your back and slide your left leg toward your body so that the knee is bent at about a 90-degree angle. Cross your right ankle over your bent knee. Grab your left thigh with both hands and slowly pull it toward you until you feel a stretch. Hold, then release.

Triangle Stretch
Level: Intermediate
Stretch Time: 3-5 breaths

This stretch will work your hamstrings and calves. Stand tall with your legs slightly farther than shoulder-distance apart. Bring your arms out from your sides in a "flying" position with your palms facing down. Keep your right foot pointed forward, but turn the left toes out. Lean to the left, bending at your hips and letting your left arm rest on your thigh. Your right arm should be straight and pointing up at the ceiling.

Pilates Advanced Leg Stretch
Level: Intermediate
Stretch Time: 3-5 breaths

This stretch targets your gluteal muscles. Start by lying on your left side. Bend your left leg to support your body but keep your right leg straight. Inhale and use your core muscles to raise your right leg up as you exhale. Hold your leg in the air and take 3 breaths before you bring it back down.

Wide Leg Advanced Forward Bend
Level: Intermediate
Stretch Time: 3-5 breaths

This stretch will work your hamstrings. Stand tall with your feet farther than shoulder-width apart and your feet pointing forward. Keeping your legs straight, slowly bend forward at the hips. Keep your back flat as you bend until your hands can touch the ground. Bend your elbows to give your hamstrings a deeper stretch. Bring your head toward the floor.

Wide Leg Advanced Hamstring Stretch
Level: Intermediate
Stretch Time: 10-30 seconds

This stretch will work your hamstrings. Stand tall with your feet farther than shoulder width apart and your back straight. Twist your upper body so that it is aligned over your right foot. Bending from your waist, reach your hands toward your right foot and let your upper body come down over your leg.

Seated Cross Legged Forward Bend
Level: Beginner
Stretch Time: 10-30 seconds

This stretch targets your hamstrings. Sit down with your legs crossed, Indian style. Bend forward slightly and rest your hands in front of your legs, letting your back curve naturally. Relax your head, neck, and shoulders. Take a few deep breaths and hold this stretch for 10 to 30 seconds.

Seated Shin Stretch
Level: Beginner
Stretch Time: 10-30 seconds

This stretch targets your shins. Kneel, straightening pointing your toes to allow the tops of your feet to face the floor. Gently move your body backward to push down on your heels and stretch the front of your lower leg.

Seated Advanced Hurdler Stretch
Level: Intermediate
Stretch Time: 10-30 seconds

This stretch will stretch your hamstrings and inner thighs. Sit on the floor. Stretch your legs out forward into a "V" shape and relax your shoulders. Bend your left knee, swinging it outward and placing the bottom of your foot against your right thigh. Your upper body should face your right leg. Bend forward over your right leg and wrap your hands around your right foot.

Side Mermaid Stretch
Level: Intermediate
Stretch Time: 10-30 seconds

This will stretch your inner thighs. Kneel on the floor, lowering your hips to the right of your knees, ultimately resting on your right hip and supporting your upper body on your right arm. Lift your left arm over your head, stretching it up and to the right while simultaneously lowering your right shoulder toward your right hip.

Chapter 5: Arm and Shoulder Stretches

Your arms, which include your biceps, triceps, and forearm muscles, are an important part of your body. You use them every day to move your hands, reach for things, lift things, and gesture.

Your shoulders, which are connected to your arms, are equally important in helping you lift heavy objects and allowing you to raise your arms over your body. Your shoulders consist of the rotator cuff, the subscapularis, the scapula, the teres minor, and the deltoid muscles.

Various combinations of muscles and joints in your arms and shoulders are what enable you to make normal, everyday movements. There are a variety of stretches you can incorporate into your routine to ensure that these muscles stay strong and flexible. This chapter will be all about the different types of arm stretches you may find helpful.

Note: when a description below mentions only one side of your body, perform it on the other side as well. Your objective is to reach balanced flexibility

Triceps Stretch
Level: Beginner
Stretch Time: 10-30 seconds

Sit on a chair. Raise your right arm, bending it at the elbow behind your head so that your hand stretches down the center of your back. Use your left hand to grasp your wrist and pull it downwards until a stretch occurs in your triceps. If you cannot reach your wrist you can simply pull your arm back from below the elbow.

Biceps Stretch
Level: Beginner
Stretch Time: 10-30 seconds

Stand up and clasp your hands together behind you, interlacing your fingers. Rotate the palms until they are facing down. Straighten your arms, raising them out and up. A stretch should occur in your biceps.

Biceps Stretch Variation #1
Level: Beginner
Stretch Time: 10-30 seconds

Stand up and stretch one arm out with your palm open and your thumb pointing upwards. Position your palm on a stationary object such as a doorframe. Rotate your torso away from your arm while keeping the rest of your body stationary.

Prayer Hands Stretch
Level: Beginner
Stretch Time: 10-30 seconds

Stand straight. Hold your palms in front of you and place them together as if you were praying. Keeping your palms together, lower your hands until you feel a stretch in your forearms.

Reverse Prayer Stretch
Level: Beginner
Stretch Time: 10-30 seconds

This will stretch the backs of your forearms, along with your fingers and your wrists. Stand straight. Instead of putting your palms together, this time put the backs of your hands together. Your fingers should be pointed downwards. Raise your hands upward, with your forearms approaching a horizontal position, until a stretch occurs.

Front Shoulder Stretch
Level: Beginner
Stretch Time: 10-30 seconds

This stretch targets your front shoulder muscles. Stand tall and keep your shoulders back for this stretch. Clasp your hands together behind you. Slowly raise your arms up over your upper body until a stretch occurs.

Crossover Shoulder Stretch
Level: Beginner
Stretch Time: 10-30 seconds

This stretch targets your shoulders and deltoid muscles. Take one arm and position it across your chest, keeping it straight and your elbow locked. Use your free hand to push in on your triceps until a stretch occurs in your shoulder.

Shoulder Stretch Variation #1
Level: Beginner
Stretch Time: 10-30 seconds

This stretch will work your shoulders. Stand and extend your right arm out to the side with your palm facing forward and your thumb pointing upward. The arm should be slightly angled downward so that your hand is level with your hip. Position your right arm against the right wall past a doorframe and turn your upper body to the left until you feel a stretch in your shoulder and bicep.

Passive Internal Rotation Stretch
Level: Beginner
Stretch Time: 10-30 seconds

This stretch targets your subscapularis muscle. Stand straight, grasping a light stick – such as a yardstick or a broom handle – behind your back. Cup one end in your right hand. Grasp the stick with your left hand. Slide the stick horizontally to the left until you feel a stretch in your right shoulder. Hold, then release.

Passive External Rotation Stretch
Level: Beginner
Stretch Time: 10-30 seconds

This stretch targets your teres minor muscle. Stand, holding a light stick – such as a yardstick or a broom handle – in your hands. Hold the stick in front of you, grasping it in your left hand, and cupping the end with your right hand. Push the stick horizontally to the left until you feel a stretch in the back of your shoulder. Hold this, then release.

Sleeper Stretch
Level: Beginner
Stretch Time: 10-30 seconds

This stretch targets your teres minor muscle. Find a flat surface and lie on your right side. Slide your right arm out until it is at a 90-degree angle to your body, then bend your elbow until your forearm is vertical. Using your left arm, gently press the forearm forward, lowering the palm toward the floor until a stretch occurs in the back of your shoulder. You should not need much motion to feel a stretch.

Arm Circles
Level: Beginner
Stretch Time: 30 seconds

This is a dynamic stretch that targets your arms and your shoulder joints. Stand, with both arms straight out from your sides at shoulder level. Start swinging them back then downward in a circular motion. After you've completed 10 circles, reverse direction and make 10 more circles. You can vary the size of your circles, gradually enlarging them until your hands swing past your hips and over your head, then reducing the size until they are back to small movements near the horizontal.

Pronated Arm Swings
Level: Intermediate
Stretch Time: 30 seconds

This stretch targets your arm muscles in general. Attach weights to your wrists. Stand with your arms at your sides, with your palms facing forward. Swing both arms out away from your sides. As your arms near shoulder height, turn your thumbs downward and let your arms swing down behind your back.

Scissor Stretch
Level: Intermediate
Stretch Time: 30 seconds

This stretch targets the muscles that enable you to pull your arms toward your body while it flexes the joints in your elbow. Stand up and hold your arms out to your sides with your palms facing the floor Swing your arms horizontally forward across your chest, crossing your left arm over your right. Reverse direction, separating both arms and swinging them back past the starting position to behind your shoulders. Swing them forward a second time, crossing your right arm over your left, then back as before.

Lying Front Deltoid Stretch
Level: Intermediate
Stretch Time 10-30 seconds

This stretch targets your anterior deltoid muscles. Sit on the floor and lean back, placing your arms behind you with your fingers pointed behind your body. Slowly slide your hips forward until you feel the stretch in your arms.

Bound Lotus Shoulder Stretch
Level: Advanced
Stretch Time: 10-30 seconds

This stretch will work your shoulders. Stand tall. Reach your right hand behind your waist. Place the fingers of that hand into the palm of your left hand. Pull the right hand forward to stretch the front of your shoulder. Repeat for the other shoulder.

Lotus Arm Standing Stretch
Level: Advanced
Stretch Time: 10-30 seconds

This stretch will work the back of your shoulder. Stand tall. Bend the elbow of your right arm and reach your right arm across your body, placing your right hand on your left shoulder. Your right elbow will be pointing forward beneath your chin. Keeping your head and neck straight, use your left arm to pull your right elbow toward the left shoulder, while allowing your right shoulder blade to move outward.

One-Armed Swastikasana Stretch
Level: Advanced
Stretch Time: 10-30 seconds

This stretch will involve your arms and shoulders. Lie on your stomach. Stretch your right arm out perpendicular to your body with your palm down. Inhale.

This stretch targets your middle back. Sit in a chair. Make a slight right turn and position your right arm on the arm rest. Place your other hand on the front of the other arm rest. Keep your hips aligned with your legs and slowly rotate your upper body to the right and forward. Hold the stretch, then release. After several repetitions switch sides and repeat to the left.

Sitting Side Bends
Level: Beginner
Stretch Time: 10 seconds

This stretch targets your upper back. Sit on the floor. Place your hands behind your head. Without leaning forward, slowly bend to the right until you feel the stretch in your back.

Knee Drops
Level: Beginner
Stretch Time: 10-30 seconds

This stretch will work your lower back. Lie on the floor. Raise your legs up and bend your knees at a 90 degree angle. Extend your arms on the floor out to your sides for stability. Straighten your legs, lowering them slowly to right before they touch the floor and hold them there. Then raise your legs back to the starting position.

Toe Touches
Level: Beginner
Stretch Time: 10 seconds

This stretch targets your middle back. Begin by sitting in a chair. Keeping your back straight, bend your upper body and use both hands to touch your toes. Come back up. As you practice this stretch you can make it more challenging by extending your feet further to increase your stretching distance.

Exercise Ball Stretch
Level: Intermediate
Stretch Time: 10-30 seconds

This stretch targets your upper back and requires an exercise ball. Sit down on the ball. Gently roll your body backward until the back of your legs touch the ball. Then roll forward to the starting position.

Cat/Cow Stretch
Level: Advanced
Stretch Time: 15-30 seconds

This exercise will stretch your spine, and your hips. Get down on your hands and knees. Keep your palms flat and spread your fingers. Your back should be flat, with your head, neck and back parallel. Inhale, looking up as you draw your shoulders back and tilting your hips to allow your back to sway downwards. Hold this position, then exhale as you drop your head and tighten your abdomen, rounding your back upward.

Elbow Tuck
Level: Intermediate
Stretch Time: 15-30 seconds
This stretch targets your middle back. Stand up and place your hands behind your back, clasping them together. Pull your elbows back and together as close as you can while you look up and stretch your head and shoulders backward to supplement the stretch.

Single Leg Glute Stretch
Level: Intermediate
Stretch Time: 10-30 seconds

This stretch will work your lower back. Lie down on the floor. Lift your right knee and move it toward your chest, angling it toward your left shoulder. Pull on the back of your knee with both hands until a stretch occurs.

Prayer Lunge Stretch
Level: Advanced
Stretch Time: 10-30 seconds

This stretch targets your lower back. Stand with your feet shoulder-width apart. Keep your arms close to your body. Raise your elbows to your shoulders and tighten your abdomen muscles. Clench your fists and bring your hands together in front of you. Step your left leg at least one foot forward and gently bend your knees into a squat. Keep your left foot flat and divide your weight between it and the bent toes of your foot. Maintain straight posture in your upper body during this stretch.

Fists Forward Bend
Level: Intermediate
Stretch Time: 15-30 seconds

This stretch targets your entire spine. Stand with your feet shoulder-width apart. Bend your knees and let your upper body bend over your legs until your stomach touches your thighs. Ball each hand into a fist and position them in the opposite creases of your elbows. Squeeze your fists as you relax your head, back, and neck.

Downward Facing Dog
Level: Advanced
Stretch Time: 5 to 10 breaths

This stretch targets your spine and lower back. Get down on all fours. Inhale as you relax your upper back and straighten your elbows. Exhale, extending your hips upward, and straightening your legs to form an upside down "V" shape. Relax your head and let it hang down between your arms.

Chapter 7: Hip Stretches

Your hips, like your legs, are responsible for much of your mobility. They allow you to walk, run, and jump. They are responsible for carrying the entire weight of your upper body.

Your hip joint consists of your pelvic bone and your thigh bones. Your hip muscles consist of flexors, adductors, extensors, and rotators. Although your hips are pretty durable, they are not indestructible. As you age and place more wear and tear on them, your chances of injuring or breaking your hips can increase. Many seniors suffer from hip injuries. By stretching your hips every day, you can help them work as long as possible.

Note: when a description below mentions only one side of your body, perform it on the other side as well. Your objective is to reach balanced flexibility

Butterfly Stretch
Level: Beginner
Stretch Time: 10-30 seconds

This stretch targets your inner thighs, hip flexors, and your groin. Sit in a cross-legged position. Place the bottoms of your feet together with your heels about two feet in front of your torso. Slowly press your arms down on your legs to stretch them gently apart. You can optionally choose to lean forward for a more advanced stretch.

Extended Wide Squat
Level: Intermediate
Stretch Time: 5 breaths

This stretch opens up both hips and also targets your lower back. **Stand, with your feet more than shoulder width apart.** Bend your knees and lower your hips to the ground. Bring your palms together and press your elbows against the inside of your knees to open your hips even further. Take 5 breaths, then bring your hands in contact with the floor and walk them backwards until a stretch occurs.

Happy Baby Stretch
Level: Beginner
Stretch Time: 10-30 seconds

This stretch will work your hip flexors. Lie down on the floor and bend your knees over your upper body like a baby. Use both hands to grasp your feet between your knees and feel the stretch.

Internal Hip Rotator Stretch

Level: Beginner
Stretch Time: 10-30 seconds

This stretch will work your hip rotators. Sit on the floor. Cross your left leg over your right leg and press your hand down on your left thigh. Once you feel resistance breathe out and tilt your hips forward. Repeat the stretch for the opposite leg.

External Hip Rotator Stretch
Level: Beginner
Stretch Time: 10-30 seconds

This stretch will work your hip rotators. Start by sitting down on the floor. Cross your left leg over the right. Use two hands to grasp your left knee and pull it toward your right shoulder. Breathe out as you pull it up to the point of resistance. Hold this position for 30 seconds. Repeat with the right knee.

Head to Knee Stretch
Level: Advanced
Stretch Time: 10-30 seconds

This stretch involves your hip flexors. Sit on the floor and straighten out your legs before you. Breathe in and bend your left knee, putting the sole of your left foot against the top of your right inner thigh. Keeping both hips firmly on the floor, breathe in as you reach your right arm straight up and then forward and let it land naturally on your right leg. Slowly bend your right shoulder down toward your right knee, allowing your right elbow to lower to the floor inside your leg until you feel a stretch.

Deep Squat Hip Stretch
Level: Intermediate
Stretch Time: 2 seconds

This stretch targets your pelvic muscles. **Stand with your feet shoulder-width apart.** Bend down and hold your toes. Drop your body down into a deep squat without bending your arms. Continue to hold your toes and then raise your hips up and straighten your knees.

Floor Hip Stretch #1
Level: Intermediate
Stretch Time: 10-30 seconds

This stretch targets your hip rotators. Lie on your back, bend your right knee as you plant the sole of your right foot on the floor. Cross your left leg over the right knee at the ankle. Without lifting your head, tighten your abdomen, press your lower back into the floor, and raise your right foot off the floor. Use your right hand to steady your ankle as you gently press down with your left hand on your left knee, flexing the hip open.

Low Lunge
Level: Advanced
Stretch Time: 5 breaths

This stretch targets your hips. Begin in the downward facing dog position. From this position, slide your left foot forward to between your hands while you lower your right knee to the floor. Release your hands from the floor and raise your head and torso to a vertical position. Tilting the bottom of your pelvis forward should cause your spine to lengthen. Take 5 breaths in this position.

High Lunge
Level: Advanced
Stretch Time: 5 breaths

This stretch targets your hips. Assume a downward facing dog position. From there, slide your left foot in between your hands and lift your hands from the floor, raising your torso until you are standing with head upright, in a lunge position, keeping square hips and gently tucking in your tailbone. Press both heels into the ground.

Short Adductor Stretch
Level: Beginner
Stretch Time: 10 seconds

This stretch targets your hip adductors. Get down on your left knee, with your right leg making a right angle in front of it. Breathe in and move your right foot a few inches to the right. Breathe out and lean toward your right knee Hold this position for 10 seconds. Back off and move your foot to the right again before repeating the stretch (don't forget to breathe). Do this several times, as you expand the distance to the right.

Long Adductor Stretch
Level: Beginner
Stretch Time: 10 seconds

This stretch targets your hip adductors. Again, get down on your left knee, but this time extend your right leg straight out, slightly right of center. Lean forward and use both hands to stabilize yourself as you lower your hips to feel the stretch. Hold for a few seconds, then back off and angle your leg a little farther to the right before sinking down to stretch again.

Lizard Pose Stretch
Level: Advanced
Stretch Time: 10 seconds

This stretch targets your hip flexors. Assume a downward facing dog position. From there, lunge your right leg forward. Press your forearms on the floor next to your right leg, careful not to move your left leg. Hold this position for 10 seconds.

Warrior Pose Stretch
Level: Advanced
Stretch Time: 5 breaths

This stretch targets your hips and pelvic muscles. Stand in a wide lunge position with your right leg forward and bent at a 90 degree angle. Ensure that your knee is positioned directly over the foot. Turn your left foot out for balance and allow your upper body to face toward the left. Inhale deeply. As you exhale, lower your right shoulder to the front side of your right leg. Take 5 breaths as you hold this position.

Frog Pose Stretch
Level: Advanced
Stretch Time:

This stretch targets your hip flexors. Get down on your hands and knees with your forearms on the ground. Widen your knees as far as you can, moving one at a time, and keep them bent so that your thighs are positioned at a 90-degree angle. Flex your feet. Keep your ribs in and your tailbone tucked under. Breathe in and out and feel your hips open.

Kneeling Hip Stretch
Level: Beginner
Stretch Time: 10-30 seconds

This stretch targets your hip flexors. Get down on your right knee. Your left knee should be bent and aligned over your left ankle. Move your hips forward until you feel tension in your right thigh. Raise your arms over your head, keeping your elbows close and your palms facing each other. Hold this position for 30 seconds.

Seated Straddle Stretch
Level: Intermediate
Stretch Time: 5 seconds

This stretch targets your hips. Sit on the floor. Spread your feet 3 feet apart from each other. Reach your arms back, one at a time, and flatten your rear on the floor to help stretch your pelvic muscles. Sit upright and raise your head upward, away from your hips. Draw in your abdomen and ribs. Fold the top half of your body forward while bringing your hands down your legs until you feel the stretch.

Standing Hamstring Stretch
Level: Beginner
Stretch Time: 10-30 seconds

This stretch targets your hip extensors. Stand in front of a chair. Place your right foot on the chair and bend forward until a stretch occurs in the back of your left leg.

Chapter 8: Neck

Your neck begins your spinal column. Your spinal column protects your spinal cord, which connects your brain and the rest of your body. Your neck also allows you to look at things above and below your eye-level as well as things all around. Your neck can become stiff due to inactivity or sleeping on it in an odd position. In this chapter, you will learn some of the simplest stretches to ensure a pain-free neck.

Note: when a description below mentions only one side of your body, complete it on the other side as well. Your objective is to reach balanced flexibility

Chin to Chest Stretch
Level: Beginner
Stretch Time: 20-30 seconds

This stretch targets your flexion muscle. Start by looking straight ahead. Tilt your head forward and touch your chin to your neck.

Shoulder Shrugs
Level: Beginner
Stretch Time: 4 seconds per shrug

This stretch helps your shoulders and neck relax through a technique known as "Progressive Muscle Relaxation." Shrug your shoulders to your ears and hold the position for 4 seconds. Continuing the shoulder shrug, turn your hands so that the palms face forward. This will start your shoulders rolling back. Continue rolling your shoulders backward as far as they will move, then relax and let your shoulders and arms hang naturally. Repeat this stretch 10 times.

Eyes to Ceiling Stretch
Level: Beginner
Stretch Time: 20-30 seconds

This stretch targets your splenius capitus muscle. Sit down and begin with your neck centered and your eyes looking forward. Carefully bend your neck backward until you're looking at the ceiling and a stretch occurs in the front of your neck.

Upper Back Stretch
Level: Beginner
Stretch Time: 20-30 seconds

This stretch will affect the muscles of your neck and upper back. Stand tall with your arms crossed before you at the wrists. Raise your arms until they are straight above your head. Hold the stretch, then release.

Levator Scapulae Stretch
Level: Beginner
Stretch Time: 30 seconds

This stretch targets your levator scapulae muscles. Stand straight and place your left straight arm slightly behind your left hip with the back of your hand resting against the hip. This is also called the pocket stretch because you next move your head to look at your right pants pocket. To add a little deeper stretch, place the fingers of your right hand over your head on the back left corner of your skull, using only the weight of your hand to increase the stretch.

Side to Side Stretch
Level: Beginner
Stretch Time: 20-30 seconds

This stretch targets the neck muscles that enable you to rotate your head. Sit straight on a chair and begin with your head facing straight forward. Slowly turn your head to the right and look over your shoulder until you feel a stretch occur. Hold for 30 seconds, then return slowly to the starting position and repeat the process to the left. As you rotate your head, do not tilt it, but keep it on an even horizontal swivel.

Corner Stretch
Level: Beginner
Stretch Time: 20-30 seconds

This stretch targets your neck, chest, and shoulder muscles. Stand facing a corner, about two feet back. Keep your feet together and position your forearms up against each wall. Your elbows should be a little below your shoulders. Lean into the corner until a stretch occurs. Hold this stretch for 20 to 30 seconds.

Behind the Back Stretch
Level: Beginner
Stretch Time: 10-30 seconds

This stretch works the sides of your neck. Stand with your feet hip-width apart. Place your arms behind your back. Grasp your left arm with your right hand and pull both down and away from your back. As you do this, tilt your head to the left, approaching your shoulder with your left ear. After holding this stretch, release it and repeat on the right side of your body.

Ear to Shoulder Stretch
Level: Beginner
Stretch Time: 20-30 seconds

This stretch targets your lateral flexion muscles. Begin by looking straight forward. Slowly tilt your head to the left, attempting to touch your shoulder with your left ear. When you feel the stretch on the right side of your neck, hold this stretch for 20 to 30 seconds.

Seated Neck Release
Level: Beginner
Stretch Time: 20 seconds

This stretch targets the sides of your neck. Sit down in a chair with your face straight forward. Drop your right arm to the right side of the chair, bending your fingers to grasp the edge of the chair. Use your left hand to gently tilt your head to the left. You can apply light pressure until you feel a slight stretch in the right side of your neck.

Neck Extensor Stretch
Level: Beginner
Stretch Time: 10-30 seconds

This stretch targets the neck extensor and the suboccipital muscles. Sit in a straight chair with your shoulders above your hips and your eyes looking straight ahead. Slowly press your head straight backward as you keep your gaze straight ahead. Your chin will seemingly tuck against your neck, but your head will not tip at all. Hold this stretch, feeling the pull down either side of your spine that begins at your neck.

Chapter 9: Chest

Your chest houses your heart, lungs, and other vital organs. The muscles of your chest include your pectoralis major and the pectoralis minor. The pectoralis major is what pulls your arm forward across your chest, while the pectoralis minor muscles allow you to move your shoulders forward. Like your neck, there are a few simple stretches you can perform to ensure that your chest muscles stay stretched out and flexible.

Note: when a description below mentions only one side of your body, perform it on the other side as well. Your objective is to reach balanced flexibility

Wide Arm Stretch
Level: Beginner

This stretch works your pectoralis major and pectoralis minor muscles. Stand straight with your feet shoulder width apart and your chest high. Extend both arms straight out from your sides with your palms facing the floor. Move your arms as far back as you can until a stretch occurs in your chest. Hold this stretch for 30 seconds and return to the starting position.

Pointed Elbow Stretch
Level: Beginner
Stretch Time: 10-30 seconds

This stretch targets your pectoralis major and minor. Stand tall and place your hands against your lower back. Bend your elbows backwards until a stretch occurs. Hold this stretch for 30 seconds and return to your starting position.

Hands Behind Head
Level: Beginner
Stretch Time: 10-30 seconds

This stretch targets both pectoralis major and pectoralis minor muscles. Stand with your feet shoulder-width apart. Weave your fingers together behind your head. Your elbows should be pointed out to your sides. Squeeze your elbows backward as far as you can. Your head should not move during this stretch. Hold this position for 30 seconds.

Door Stretch
Level: Beginner
Stretch Time: 10-30 seconds

Stand just behind an open doorway with your feet shoulder width apart. Raise your right arm out from your side, placing your right forearm vertically outside the right side of the doorway. Your right elbow should be slightly above the shoulder. Keeping your torso vertical, step forward with your right leg into the doorway. As your right arm is pressed backward you should feel a stretch to your chest. Repeat this process with your left arm.

Camel Pose Stretch
Level: Advanced
Stretch Time: 5 breaths

This stretch works your chest muscles. Get down on your knees and keep them at least two fist widths apart. Place your hands on your lower back. Tighten your abdomen and tip your tailbone down. Gazing toward the far wall, lift your chest up and squeeze your shoulder blades together. Hold this stretch for five breaths.

Bridge Pose Stretch
Level: Advanced
Stretch Time: 5 breaths

This stretch targets your pectoralis major and pectoralis minor muscles. Lie down on your back. Bend your knees and place your feet on the floor with your heels against your hips. Placing your hands by your sides for stability, raise your hips off the floor. As your hips rise, lift your chest also keeping your back straight. Hold for 5 breaths, then relax.

Chapter 10: Hands

Could you imagine life without your hands? With your hands you grab, clasp, and manipulate objects, and that's just for starters. Your hands have two types of muscles, extrinsic and intrinsic muscles. The extrinsic muscles enable you to forcefully grip objects while your intrinsic muscles give you the ability to perform fine motor functions. In what follows, you will find plenty of ways to stretch these muscles.

Note: when a description below mentions only one side of your body, complete it on the other side as well. Your objective is to reach balanced flexibility

Extended Arm Stretch
Level: Beginner
Stretch Time: 10-30 seconds

This stretch works your wrists and your fingers. Stand tall and stretch out your right arm in front of you with your palm facing downward. Relax your wrist, letting your fingers drop downward. Use your left hand to grasp these fingers and gently pull them back toward your body.

Clutching Stretch
Level: Beginner
Stretch Time: 10 seconds

This stretch targets your finger muscles and helps prevent them from getting sore after constant typing or holding a small object – such as a pencil – for a long period of time. Start by spreading apart the fingers of each hand. Keeping your wrists straight, bend your fingers at only the first two knuckles so that your fingertips point back toward your arm. Hold your fingers in this stretch for 10 seconds, then release.

Desk Press Stretch
Level: Beginner
Stretch Time: 10 seconds

This stretch targets your wrists and elbows. Sit in front of a flat surface such as a desk. Position your palms face up beneath the surface and press upwards. Hold this position for 10 seconds.

Prayer Press Stretch
Level: Beginner
Stretch Time: 10 seconds

This stretch targets your wrists and your palms. Press your hands against each other as if you were praying. Lower your hands gently until you feel a stretch.

Ball Squeeze Stretch
Level: Beginner
Stretch Time: 5-10 seconds

This stretch strengthens your wrists. Firmly squeeze a ball for a few seconds, then release.

Finger Pulls
Level: Beginner
Stretch Time: 2 seconds

This stretch targets your fingers and helps prevent strain from overuse. Spread the fingers of your right hand. With your left hand, grasp the tip of one finger. Gently pull the fingertip up, down, and from side to side. Repeat this for each finger; then switch hands.

Thumb Pulls
Level: Beginner
Stretch Time: 10 seconds

This stretch targets your thumbs. Fold your hand into the "thumbs up" position. Use your free hand to gently stretch your thumb backward toward your body.

Thumb Pushes
Level: Beginner
Stretch Time: 10 seconds

This stretch targets your thumbs. Fold your hand into the "thumbs up" position. While trying to hold your thumb still, use your free hand to push your thumb forward. Hold this position for 10 seconds.

Open and Close Stretch
Level: Beginner
Stretch Time: 10-20 times per hand

This stretch targets your entire hand and helps you maintain mobility. Simply ball your hand into a fist and then open your hand as wide as you can.

Finger Spread Stretch
Level: Beginner
Stretch Time: 10-20 times per hand

This stretch targets your fingers. Without bending your wrists, bring your straight fingers together. Spread your fingers apart and then bring them back together. Repeat this stretch 10 to 20 times.

Thumb Spread Stretch
Level: Beginner
Stretch Time: 10-20 times per hand
This stretch targets your thumb and imitates the finger spread stretch. Simply hold your thumb in towards your index finger and then pull it away while keeping your wrist straight. Repeat this stretch 10 to 20 times.

Overhead Reach Stretch
Level: Beginner
Stretch Time: 10-30 seconds

This stretch targets your hands and forearms. Interlace your fingers, turn your palms out, and stretch your arms above your head.

Figure 8 Stretch
Level: Beginner
Stretch Time: 10-15 seconds

This stretch involves your wrists, your forearms, and your fingers. Hold your elbows against your sides with each hand in a soft fist. Keeping your elbows against your sides, move your wrists in a figure eight motion. Continue this motion for 10 to 15 seconds, then rest and repeat.

Chapter 11: Full Body Stretches

Note: when a description below mentions only one side of your body, perform it on the other side as well. Your objective is to reach balanced flexibility

Runner's Stretch

Stand straight and inhale. Exhale as you step forward with your right foot into a lunge position and lower your body until your fingers can make contact with the ground. Inhale as you straighten out your right leg. Exhale as you slowly return to the lunge position and then back to your starting position. Repeat this stretch 4 times on each leg.

Full Body Exercise Ball Stretch

This stretch requires an exercise ball. Start by sitting on the ball, with your feet apart for stability. Roll the ball slightly forward as you lie backward atop it, keeping your legs fairly straight and spread apart enough to keep your body stable. Reach your hands over your head and feel the total body stretch. Allow your whole body to luxuriate in this stretch for 15 to 30 seconds.

Standing Side Stretch

Stand straight with your feet fairly close together. Reach your arms over your head, interlacing your fingers. Breathe in and reach upward. Breathe out and slowly bend your body to the right. Take 5 deep breaths, allowing your body to stretch further each time as you exhale. Then stretch straight up. Repeat this stretch to the left.

Downward Facing Dog

Get down on your hands and knees. Inhale as you relax your upper back and look up. Exhale, straightening your knees and bringing your hips backwards to form an upside down "V" with your body Relax your head and let it hang down between your arms. Hold this stretch for ten breaths.

Forward Hang Stretch

Stand with your feet hip distance apart and your knees slightly bent. Put your hands behind your back and interlace your fingers. Inhale and stretch your arms back and up. Breathe out and bend your upper body at your waist, keeping your back straight until your back is horizontal with the floor. Hold this position for 5 deep breaths.

Plank Stretch

Begin in a push-up stance. Keep your hands directly beneath your shoulders. Press up through your hips and stretch your tailbone as your spine and hips stay level. Look straight ahead and take 5 deep breaths.

Low Lunge Arch Stretch

Begin in a lunge position with your right leg forward. Position your arms in front of your right knee and connect your hands by hooking your thumbs together. Breathe in and reach your arms up until a comfortable stretch occurs. Take 5 deep breaths.

Wheel Stretch

Lie flat on your back and pull your heels close to your hips. Bend your elbows up and spread your palms flat on the floor next to your ears. Press into the floor with your feet and raise your tailbone, careful not to completely lock your hips. Press your arms into the floor until your back arches. Allow your head to hang from your neck as your body takes a nearly circular shape. Take 5 deep breaths.

Seated Back Twist Stretch

Sit on the floor and stretch your legs in front of you. Cross your right leg over the left and set your foot down to the left of the left knee. Place your right hand flat on the ground next to your hips. Bend your left elbow and place it against your right knee for support. Breathe in and turn your upper body to the right. Exhale as you complete the twist. Look over your right shoulder and take 5 deep breaths.

Bound Angle Stretch

Sit on the floor with your hips atop a folded blanket. Place the soles of your feet together and lower your knees as close to the ground as possible, encouraging your inner thighs to relax, and allowing the legs to approach the floor. Touch the floor to each side with your fingertips, encouraging your torso to stretch straight up as you inhale. As you exhale, keep your back straight as you bend forward from the hips. Move your arms forward to support the weight of your torso as you stretch forward. Continue to stretch for 5 deep breaths.

- Elbow Tuck
- Toe Touches
- Rotations
- Spine Twist
- Cat/Cow Stretch
- Sitting Side Bends
- Exercise Ball Stretch

Hips: Unless otherwise stated, complete 3 repetitions of 20 seconds each for both sides of the body.

- Seated Straddle Stretch
- Kneeling Hip Flexor Stretch
- Frog Pose Stretch
- Long Adductor Stretch
- Short Adductor Stretch
- Floor Hip Stretch #2
- High Lunge

Neck: Unless otherwise stated, complete three repetitions of 30 seconds each for each side of the body.

- Side to Side Stretch
- Corner Stretch
- Ear to Shoulder Stretch
- Neck Extensor Stretch
- Seated Neck Release –

Chest: Unless otherwise stated, complete 3 repetitions of 5 breaths each, for both sides of the body.

- Wide Arm Stretch
- Pointed Elbow Stretch
- Hands Behind Head
- Towel Rotation Stretch
- Camel Pose Stretch
- Bridge Pose Stretch

Hands: Unless otherwise stated, complete 3 repetitions of 10 seconds each for each side of the body.

- Extended Arm Stretch
- Desk Press Stretch
- Ball Squeeze Stretch
- Finger Pulls
- Finger Spread Stretch

Advanced Stretching Routine

Legs:

- Three quadriceps stretches
- Three hamstring stretches
- Three calve stretches
- Two inner thigh stretches
- Two glute stretches

Arms and Shoulders:

- Two biceps stretches
- Two triceps stretches

- Three shoulder stretches

Back:

- Two lower back stretches
- Two middle back stretches
- Two upper back stretches
- Two spine stretches
- One full back stretch

Hips:

- Three flexor stretches
- Two adductor stretches
- Two hip rotator stretches
- Two pelvic muscle stretches
- One hip extensor stretch

Neck:

- One full set of neck stretches

Chest:

- One full set of chest stretches

Hands:

- 3 to 4 hand stretches of your choice

Full Body:

- One full set of body stretches

Sample Advanced Stretching Routine

Legs: Unless otherwise stated, complete 4 repetitions of 30 seconds each for each leg.

- Standing Quadriceps Stretch
- Side Quadriceps Stretch
- Prone Quadriceps Stretch
- Hamstring Variation #2
- Wide Leg Advanced Hamstring Stretch
- Wide Leg Advanced Forward Bend
- Calf Stretch Variation #1
- Triangle Stretch
- Seated Shin Stretch
- Seated Advanced Hurdler Stretch
- Seated Advanced Hurdler Stretch
- Glute Stretch
- Pilates Advanced Leg Stretch

Arms and Shoulders: Unless otherwise specified, complete 4 repetitions of 30 seconds each for each arm.

- Biceps Stretch
- Advanced Biceps Stretch
- Triceps Stretch
- One-Armed Swastikasana Stretch
- Front Shoulder Stretch
- Lotus Arm Standing Stretch
- Bound Lotus Shoulder Stretch

Back: Unless otherwise specified, complete 4 repetitions of 30 seconds each for each side of the body.

- Downward Facing Dog – Perform 3 repetitions of 5 breaths each
- Prayer Lunge Stretch
- Elbow Tuck
- Toe Touches
- Exercise Ball Stretch
- Sitting Side Bends
- Fists Forward Bend
- Cat/Cow Stretch

Hips: Unless otherwise specified, complete 4 repetitions of 30 seconds each for both sides of the body.

- Happy Baby Stretch
- Kneeling Hip Flexor Stretch
- Frog Pose Stretch – 3 repetitions of 5 breaths each
- Short Adductor Stretch
- Long Adductor Stretch
- Floor Hip Stretch #1
- External Hip Rotator Stretch
- Standing Hamstring Stretch
- Deep Squat Hip Stretch
- Warrior Pose Stretch – 3 repetitions of 5 breaths for each side
- Seated Straddle Stretch

Neck: Unless otherwise specified, complete 4 repetitions of 20 seconds each, for both sides of the body.

- Chin to Chest Stretch
- Shoulder Shrugs
- Eyes to Ceiling Stretch
- Levator Scapulae Stretch –
- Side to Side Stretch
- Corner Stretch
- Behind the Back Stretch
- Ear to Shoulder Stretch
- Seated Neck Release
- Neck Extensor Stretch

Chest: Unless otherwise specified complete 4 repetitions of 20 seconds each, for both sides of the body as applicable.

- Bridge Pose Stretch – 3 repetitions of 5 breaths each
- Camel Pose Stretch – 3 repetitions of 5 breaths each
- Towel Rotation Stretch
- Hands Behind Head
- Pointed Elbow Stretch
- Wide Arm Stretch
- Hand Stretches:
- Figure 8 Stretch
- Overhead Reach Stretch
- Thumb Spread Stretch
- Finger Spread Stretch

- Prayer Press Stretch

Full Body: Unless otherwise specified, complete one repetition of 5 breaths each, for both sides of the body.

- Runner's Stretch
- Full Body Exercise Ball Stretch
- Standing Side Stretch
- Forward Hang Stretch
- Plank Stretch
- Low Lunge Arch Stretch
- Wheel Stretch
- Seated Back Twist Stretch
- Bound Angle Stretch

Chapter 13: Creating Your Own Stretching Routine

Step 1: Carve out Space in Your Life

To make stretching a part of your life, the first step is to establish a location. Since stretching is so straightforward, requiring little to no equipment, it shouldn't be too hard to settle on a good place. Personally, I like to stretch in my office, where I can listen to background music and relax by myself. Another good places to stretch is any area of your house that offers enough floor space to stand, sit, and lie down.

Alternatively, a gym, which usually has designated areas for stretching will work. Weather permitting, you can also stretch outside in your backyard, on the beach, in a park, or any other favorite area. One of the beauties of picking a spot to stretch is that you don't have to visit the same place every day; you can switch it up whenever you're in the mood for a change of scenery.

Next, you'll want to settle on a stretching schedule. Which days should you stretch? Research suggests that the minimum amount of time you should spend stretching is three times a week with 30 seconds "at a stretch." However, it is acceptable to stretch for up to 6 days a week. If you are looking for optimal results, start by stretching for three days a week and work your way up to a maximum of six days. I prefer to stretch on alternate days because I believe it's good to give your muscles time to recover.

You can also choose whether to stretch once, twice or three times a day, as most stretches usually require multiple repetitions. I tend to stretch once a day, doing all the repetitions at one time. Stretching three times a day can bring optimal results.

If you find it difficult to remember to stretch, you can pair stretching with another activity, or use an activity as a trigger to stretch. For example, some people stretch whenever they watch television or stretch every time they feel bored. Others use mealtimes or work breaks as a trigger to remind them to stretch.

Now that you've picked your stretching space and your stretching schedule, you're still left with the question, "Which stretches does my body need?" .

Step 2: Decide Which Areas of Your Body Need the Most Attention

You can complete a general stretch routine fairly quickly by giving equal attention to each body part. However, if you determine that one area of your body requires special attention, you'll need to allocate extra time for that area. For example, I have suffered two shoulder injuries in the past couple of years. I know that to keep those muscles strong, they require some specific targeted stretches.

Often your body will let you know when it has specific needs, so listen to it. A while back I began suffering from plantar fasciitis, although at first, all I knew was that my heel began to hurt. After research I learned that stretching is the number one treatment for this condition. I adjusted my stretching schedule to accommodate some specific stretches that target the foot and calf area. My plantar fasciitis subsided and I was saved the time and cost of a trip to the doctor, only to have him tell me to stretch!

Step 3: Gather the Equipment You Will Need

This step should be easy, considering that the most extensive equipment you may ever need will include a resistance band, an exercise ball and maybe a few weights. I use a resistance band for my foot stretches and I now use two five-pound weights when stretching my shoulders. At any rate, prevent the need to interrupt your routine by ensuring you have everything you need at hand, *before* you begin.

Make sure you have plenty of water on hand so you can stay dehydrated between stretches. Drinking water is important to help loosen your joints.

Step 3: Warm Up

Whether you're going to do a general stretching routine or something area-specific, the third step is always to warm up. As you know, it is important to do a light warm up before you start stretching any muscles. For a general routine, you can follow the dynamic warm up outlined in Chapter Three. For specific areas, check out what you need to do to warm up those muscles. For example, my shoulder stretching warm-up consists of arm circles and pendulum swings. Even as you warm up for stretching, remember to drink water; ample hydration is essential for optimum functionality.

Step 4: Pick Some Stretches to Start

When you're new to the stretching scene, it can be difficult to figure out where to begin. When I first started out, I just randomly picked some beginner stretches to try for each area of my body: legs, arms, shoulders, back, hands, neck and chest. I gave them a try, figured out which ones worked best for me, and discontinued the stretches I found too difficult to master. Now that I've established a stretching routine, I try to add in a few new stretches every couple weeks, just to keep my routine fresh and interesting. After about two weeks, I pretty much have my routine down and can focus on getting the most out of each stretch.

Do not over-stretch. Beginners should start out holding stretches for only 10 seconds and gradually work up to a more experienced level of 30 seconds at a time. Listen to your body and back off if it starts complaining.

Step 5: Tweak Your Routine

After a few weeks, you should have a pretty good idea of which stretches you're good at, which ones you enjoy doing, and which areas of your body you think will require more attention. Sometimes you'll be surprised; you may think you don't need to focus on stretching your legs, but a simple calf stretch may reveal unusual tightness in those muscles.

Once you've gotten a feel for where you are and where you think you need to be, I recommend copying some of the sample skeleton stretching routines from the previous chapter and using them as an outline on which you can hang some of your favorite stretches. Focus on a chosen routine for about a month, then review it to see what adjustments need to be made, both in which stretches you use and in their frequency or intensity. See if you can develop from a beginner to an advanced level over the course of a few months.

Don't be afraid to try new stretches; this will keep boredom at bay and will expose your body to new ways to move and flex. You will probably be surprised at how much flexibility you gain in a few weeks! The gains in strength, posture, and energy can be significant.

Conclusion

I hope this book was able to help you learn about your body, your muscles and how stretching can improve your life.

Stretching is just as important as other forms of exercise; I hope by now you have decided to incorporate stretches into your daily routine. Proper stretching will protect your muscles from future injury, make your body flexible, and increase your sense of well-being, all by performing a few strategic stretches throughout your day.

Stretching is simple and can be accomplished almost anywhere you have enough room. It requires no special equipment, so there's nothing to keep you from getting started. Some stretches can even be done at your desk or in meetings with nobody even noticing, so take advantage of your spare minutes and start stretching today. If you can find a nice relaxing place to stretch, it makes it much more enjoyable. I have a nice pier overlooking the canal at the back of my house, and that is my favorite place to go down to and stretch. It makes it much more enjoyable. I have also found that wearing headphones and listening to uplifting music makes stretching mych more enjoyable as well.

Begin small – don't overdo it at first – and build each day until you have developed a well-rounded stretching routine that balances your body's strengths into a healthy whole. Focus on tight areas and muscle groups that may need to be healed.

It won't be long before you find yourself in much improved physical condition, able to sit comfortably for longer, able to more easily perform your favorite yoga poses (if you're into yoga), and able to both exercise and play physical games more comfortably, with less danger of injury. If you want to live a long and happy life, be sure to make stretching into a healthy habit that you perform each and every day.

Finally, if you discovered at least one thing that has helped you or that you think would be beneficial to someone else, be sure to take a few seconds to easily post a quick positive review. As an author, your positive feedback is desperately needed. Your highly valuable five star reviews are like a river of golden joy flowing through a sunny forest of mighty trees and beautiful flowers! *To do your good deed in making the world a better place by helping others with your valuable insight, just leave a nice review.*

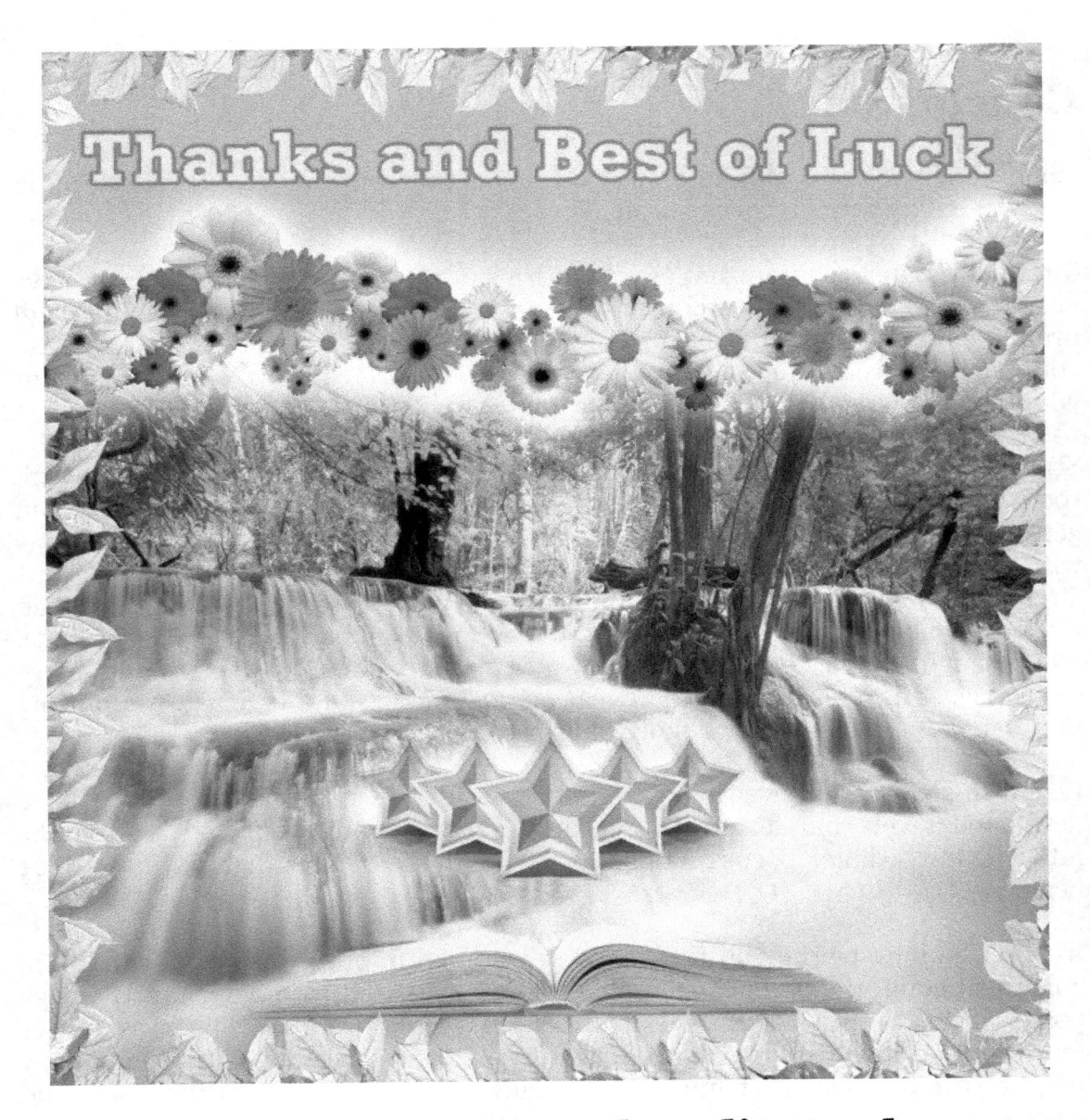

My Other Books and Audio Books
www.AcesEbooks.com

Health Books

ULTIMATE HEALTH SECRETS
HEALTH

Strategies For Dieting, Eating Healthy, Exercising, Losing Weight, The Mediterranean Diet, Strength Training, And All About Vitamins, Minerals, And Supplements

Ace McCloud

ENERGY
Ultimate Energy

Discover How To Increase Your Energy Levels Using The Best All Natural Foods, Supplements And Strategies For A Life Full Of Abundant Energy

Ace McCloud

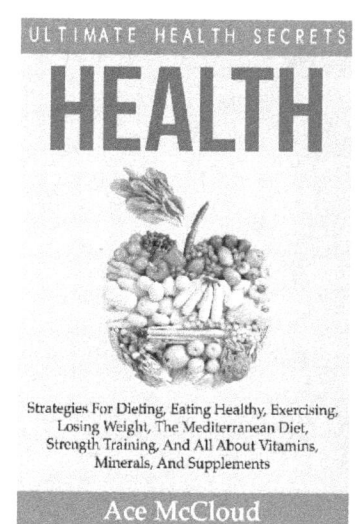

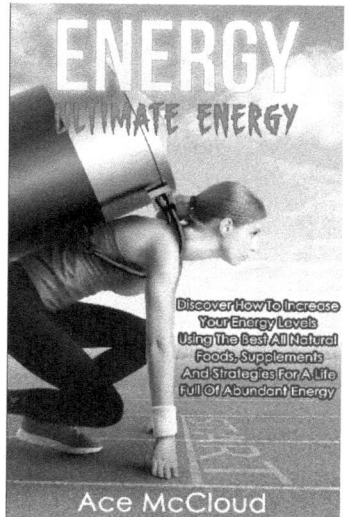

RECIPE BOOK

The Best Food Recipes That Are Delicious, Healthy, Great For Energy And Easy To Make

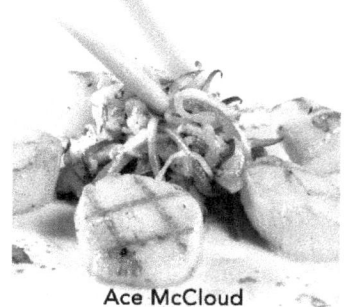

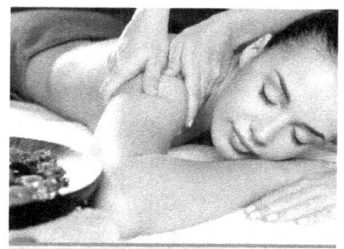

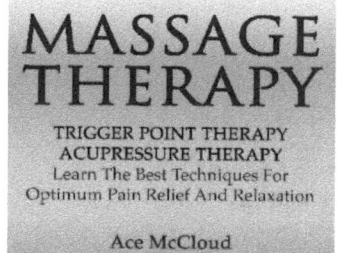

Ace McCloud

MASSAGE THERAPY

TRIGGER POINT THERAPY
ACUPRESSURE THERAPY
Learn The Best Techniques For Optimum Pain Relief And Relaxation

Ace McCloud

LOSE WEIGHT

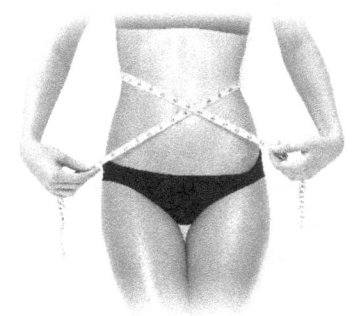

THE TOP 100 BEST WAYS TO LOSE WEIGHT QUICKLY AND HEALTHILY

Ace McCloud

FATIGUE
OVERCOME CHRONIC FATIGUE

Discover How To Energize Your Body & Mind So That You Can Bring The Energy & Passion Back Into Your Life

Ace McCloud

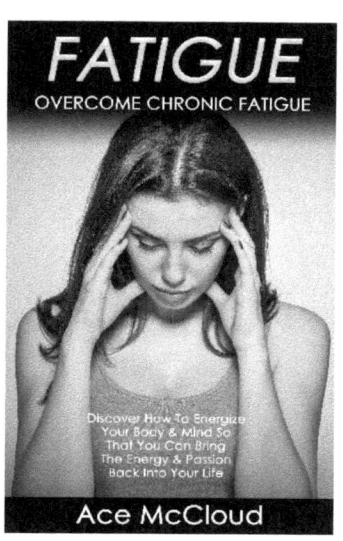

Peak Performance Books

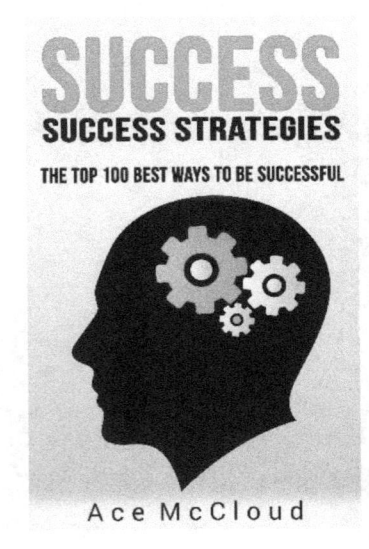

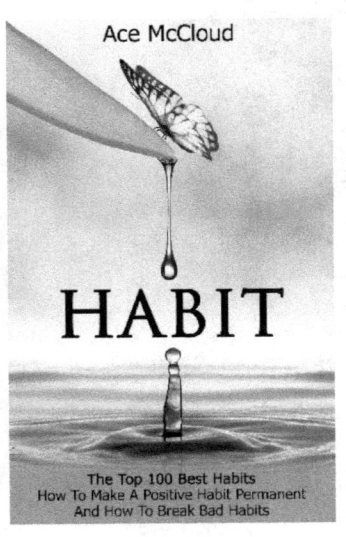

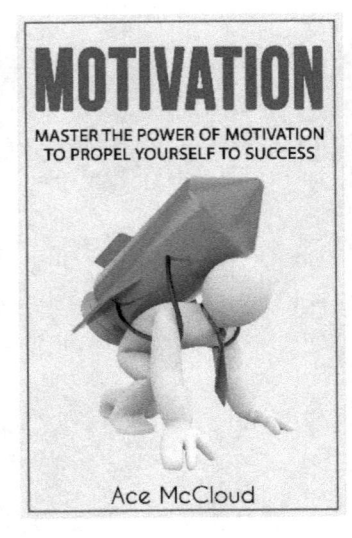

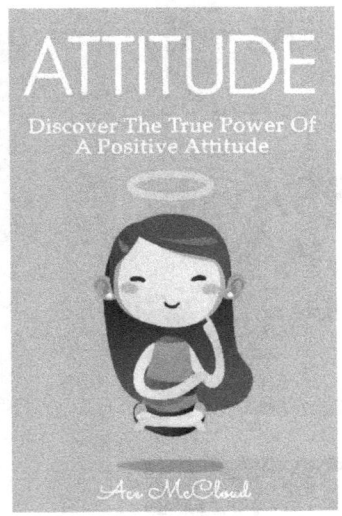

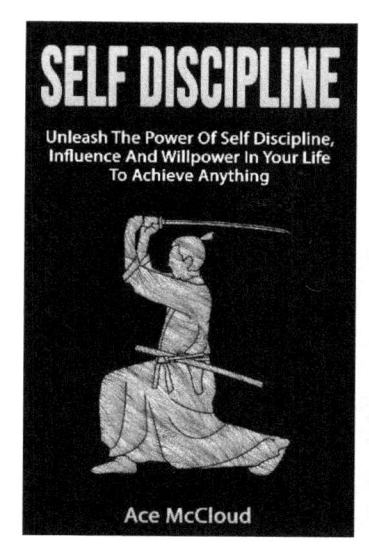

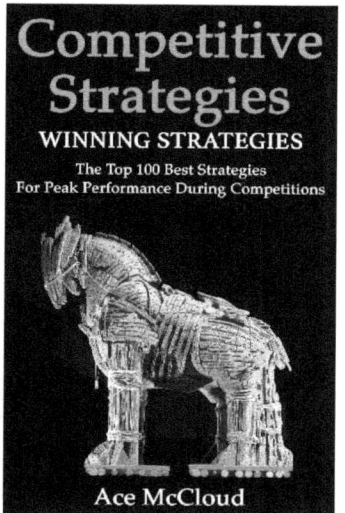

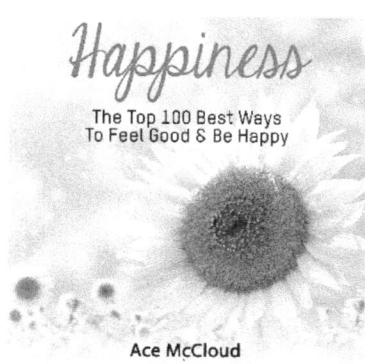

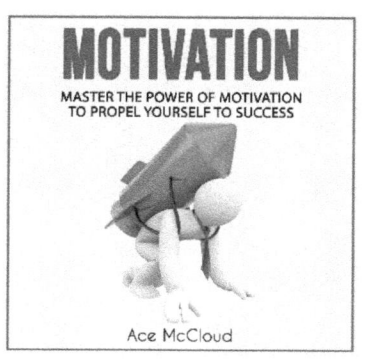

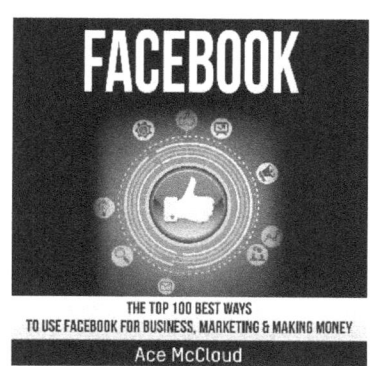

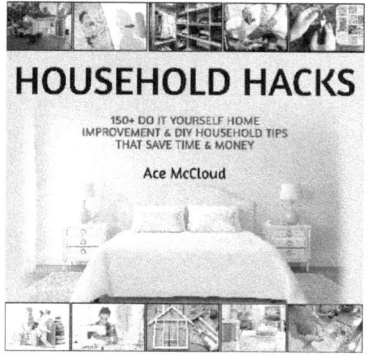

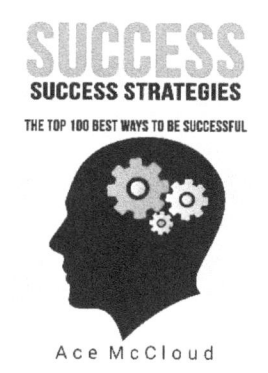

Be sure to check out my audio books as well!

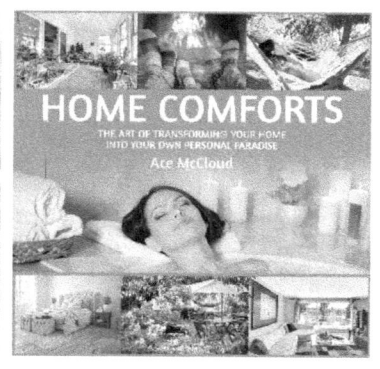

Check out my website at: **www.AcesEbooks.com** for a complete list of all of my books and high quality audio books. I enjoy bringing you the best knowledge in the world and wish you the best in using this information to make your journey through life better and more enjoyable! **Best of luck to you!**

CPSIA information can be obtained
at www.ICGtesting.com
Printed in the USA
LVHW022058100723
752064LV00009B/803